The Essential Oils Thyroid Solution

Chronic Fatigue? Weight Gain?
Brain Fog?
Get Relief with Essential Oils to
Help Heal Your Thyroid

Contents

Introduction

Immense thanks and compliments to you for purchasing this book, "The Essential Oils Thyroid Solution".
This book is a primer, for beginners, on the link between aromatherapy and thyroid healing. Are you sick and tired of losing sleep at night? Do you suffer from constant fatigue, weight gain, or inability to lose weight? Do you have inopportune (to say the least) brain fog, headaches or migraines? Other symptoms may include brittle nails, unexplained hair loss/thinning hair or always having cold hands and feet. Or do you feel depressed, anxious or irritable way more than you would like?
This book is for you if you are searching for a natural solution to your ailments and annoying symptoms. If you are looking for medical advice, a drug or prescription medicine, you may not benefit from reading this book. If you have been prescribed a thyroid medicine in order to make up for the imbalances in your hormones, yet you are still dealing with unwanted ailments or symptoms, then, as you continue to read this book you will receive valuable information for your journey to feeling like yourself again and to possibly weaning yourself off of your thyroid medicine. The thyroid is one of the most important glands in the body and about 20 million people have a thyroid issue, but only 60% of them are even aware of it!
According to research studies, a majority of people in the world are bound to suffer thyroid issues at some point in time or another in their life, due to things like diet, hereditary conditions or toxic chemical or heavy metal exposure. And women make up the majority of thyroid sufferers.
If you feel bound by your symptoms that prevent you from reaching your full potential, then it is wise to seek help and put an end to your health woes. Essential oils make for an effective, alternative solution to conventional medicine

solutions, which only treat the symptoms for thyroid issues and do not delve deep enough into the underlying causes of the condition. Presented in this book is an alternative to the conventional way of healing. Aromatherapy, the practice of using essential oils for healing, can contribute to the upkeep of good health. It could prove to be the missing link in your diet, and medication, routine and prove useful in enhancing your metabolism.

As you continue to read this book you will discover the possibilities of plant-derived medicine in your healing. Essential oils have been utilized as medicine for thousands of years and it's about time you tapped into their immeasurable potential and finally get the relief you deserve!

Check out the second book in this series, *Fermentation and Thyroid Health*, which includes over 20 delicious fermented foods recipes!

Again, thanks a million for purchasing this book; please enjoy!

Chapter 1
I Have a Butterfly in My Throat!
(or What is the Thyroid?)

We will begin by looking at the purpose of the thyroid in order to understand its function in the body. The thyroid is a part of the endocrine system. This entire system, and its organs and glands, is responsible for the release of hormones into the blood stream which are then distributed to cells and organs through the circulatory system. The thyroid is a small gland located in the front of your neck. Owing to its distinct shape, it is often referred to as the butterfly organ. It is made up of a variety of cells that have specific functions.

Despite its small size, the thyroid is larger than all the glands in the neck and it is one of the most important organs in the body. It is responsible for keeping a person's metabolism functioning optimally and produces hormones that regulate your body's metabolism. To function properly, the thyroid requires a number of processes to be in balance. If these processes and the hormones secreted from the thyroid are not in balance it can set off complications and your body will respond by trying to compensate for the imbalances.

How the Thyroid Functions

The thyroid gland and its hormones serve many different purposes in the body. The following are merely some of the functions of the thyroid gland and as you will see, it is one of the most hard working glands in the body and responsible for the maintenance of overall good health. However, an issue in the thyroid gland can lead to the development of other health issues, which will be discussed in the next chapter.

First, the boring (or fascinating, for the nerds, like me) scientific stuff...
The thyroid gland regulates production and release of thyroid hormones known as T1 (monoidothyronine), T2 (3,5-Diiodo-L-thyronine), T3 (Triiodothyronine), T4 (Thyroxine), and rT3 (Reverse Triiodothyronine). These are hormones that effect metabolism and determine how fast, or slow, your organs function including heart, brain, liver, kidneys and the digestive system. The T1 and T2 hormones are lesser known because it is still unclear what their true role is in the metabolism. This does not mean they are not important, but because there is not much known about them we will not focus on these in this book.

The T3 hormone is instrumental in raising your basal metabolic rate, as well as the consumption and use of energy and oxygen. T3 also helps with weight loss and produces serotonin in the brain (who doesn't want more of that "happiness serum"?). It also helps in maintaining a normal or ideal body temperature, with the regulating of menstrual cycles and your changing hormones and in controlling normal brain activity and enhancing the functions of the central and peripheral nervous system. The thyroid secretes the hormone called T4. Even though more T4 is produced (called T4 because each of its molecules contains 4 iodine atoms), the hormone called T3 (big surprise: T3 has 3 iodine atoms per molecule!) happens to be the most active hormone in the body as most T4 is not active and has to be converted into T3 through the bloodstream, liver or kidneys. Problems occur when T4 has difficulty being converted to T3 or when the hormones are not free, meaning they are bound to a protein in the bloodstream called thyroid binding globulin (TGB).

The hypothalamus stimulates the pituitary gland (both found in the brain) with its hormone called thyrotrophine-releasing hormone (TRH), which instructs the pituitary gland to release the thyroid stimulating hormone (TSH) or thyrotrophine. As you may be able to tell from its name, the TSH controls, i.e. stimulates, the thyroid and tells it how much or how little of its hormone it should release.

A certain type of enzymes is also involved in converting T4 to T3. These are called enzyme 5' deiodinases and they remove iodine from the hormone and help turn the thyroid hormones "on and off" and basically control and balance the hormones by controlling how much iodine is in each one. There are three different types, simply called D1, D2, and D3 and they are found in different parts of the body. The basic detail you need to know about these is that they are required for the essential conversion of T4 to T3 and there are number of causes that will impact whether they are producing properly. A few of those causes are, heavy metal toxicity, inflammation, a vast amount of cortisol, selenium deficiency and stress. D2 works in the pituitary gland and regulates the gland's T3 levels and has been said to be a thousand times more efficient in converting T4 to T3 than D1, of which a very small amount is located in the pituitary gland. D2 also reacts in a contrary way than D1 and D3 to stress, to inflammation, and to the other causes of poor conversion mentioned above. In other words, it is not inhibited by causes like stress like D1 and D3 are inhibited. Therefore, if a doctor relies only on a test that determines the levels of TSH to treat your symptoms, be skeptical.

The thyroid requires iodine, zinc, B vitamins, selenium and many other factors to function optimally. But, it is important to have a very thorough test done of all of your hormones in order to determine what is truly causing poor thyroid functioning. The good news is that eating a balanced diet, exercising, and using a therapeutic, essential oil regimen will go a long way in finding relief and healing. This book adheres to a holistic perspective in regard to the body's healing and health. Holistic ways of healing will be discussed in the coming chapters, but first we will talk about the resulting diseases caused by poor thyroid function.

Are you enjoying this book? Please leave a review!

Chapter 2
The Reasons for Your Annoying Symptoms (or Understanding Hypo and Hyperthyroidism)

Hyperthyroidism

Hyperthyroidism is a condition where there is an excess release of thyroid hormone in the body. A lower percentage of people have this, as compared to those with hypothyroidism, although if hypothyroidism is treated with too much thyroid hormone medicine, it can lead to hyperthyroidism. It is a delicate balancing act, which is one of the reasons it is recommended in this book to steer clear of synthetic medicine if at all possible and go the natural route as much as possible. Hyperthyroidism can occur if there is an excess release of the thyroxine in the body. There can be multiple effects or causes of hyperthyroidism and some are as follows.

Graves' disease
Grave's disease, the most wide-spread condition of hyperthyroidism, is a condition that can be hereditary in nature. It is offset by an overactive thyroid that produces the thyroid hormone in excess. It can lead to Graves' ophthalmopathy or skin lesions.

Multinodular goiter

Multinodular goiter refers to a condition where individual nodules or multiple nodules form in the neck thereby causing a swelling. This can prompt the thyroid gland to overproduce thyroxine.

Excess intake of medication
An excess intake of medication can also cause hyperthyroidism. Hyperthyroidism can occur if a person takes a dosage that is higher than the recommended value. Some people tend to take higher doses of thyroid medicine in an attempt to lose weight.

Overactive pituitary
If the pituitary gland turns overactive then it can lead to hyperthyroidism. An issue in the pituitary gland such as a tumor can lead to over-secretion of TSH thereby prompting the thyroid to secrete too much thyroid hormone. This can also lead to an inflammation of the thyroid gland, which is diagnosed as hyperthyroidism.

Symptoms
Tremors
Excessive sweating
Hair thinning
Rapid heart rate
Thyroid gland enlargement
Eye puffiness

These form some of the symptoms of hyperthyroidism. These can vary depending on the person and their overall health. Most people are prescribed medicines that help in controlling the amount of thyroid hormone that is secreted in the body. Radioactive iodine is also injected in some patients to help control this condition. Many thyroid patients continue to complain of symptoms despite being on medications. Thankfully, there are natural options and patients can also be administered essential oils. We will look at this in detail in the chapters to come.

Hypothyroidism

Hypothyroidism is the opposite of hyperthyroidism and results in the under functioning of the thyroid gland and a slow metabolism. Remember in the last chapter how we discussed that there can be problems if your body has a hard time converting T4 to T3? If your body cannot metabolize T4 this will result in the production of rT3, which inhibits T3 and its ability to produce results in the body. When a person is under a constant stream of stress due to different factors, like emotional trauma, extreme exercise, too little sleep or many other circumstances, this will cause the adrenals to overproduce cortisol. Cortisol is instrumental in blocking the conversion of T4 to T3. T3 and rT3 cannot coexist, therefore if there is high rT3 then there is low T3. And this is what we want to avoid, this is what causes hypothyroidism.

Possible Outcomes or Effects of Hypothyroidism
Hypothyroidism can have many effects associated with it, including:
An inflammation of the thyroid gland also known as thyroiditis. This can cause the thyroid gland to malfunction and lead to hypothyroidism
Hashimoto's is a disease where the body turns against its immune system causing an inflammation in the thyroid gland.
Congenital hypothyroidism is a condition where babies develop the disease within the womb and are born with a malfunctioning thyroid
An imbalance in the iodine levels in the body can lead to hypothyroidism

Symptoms

Hypothyroidism is sometimes hard to detect because the symptoms can be a result of other complications that are not related, but some common symptoms are as follows:
fatigue
weight gain
cognitive problems or brain fog
depression
constipation
dry skin
brittle hair
slower heart rate
high cholesterol
weakness
cold hands and feet or sensitivity to cold

These form the different symptoms of hypothyroidism. If you notice any of these then it will be best to consult a physician and begin the testing process to determine where your healing efforts should be directed.

What is Hashimoto's?

Hashimoto's is an autoimmune disease where the body turns against its own organs and starts attacking them. It begins to attack the thyroid leading to inflammation and an inability to secrete an adequate amount of thyroxine in the body.

Treatment

In many cases, conventional doctors will prescribe a synthetic thyroid replacement hormone called Synthroid, which is a T4 only treatment, meaning it will add only synthetic T4 to your body in hopes that the presence of more T4 will inherently lead to more T3. Depending on the severity of the thyroid condition, some people are also advised surgery.

According to Dr. John A. Robinson, a Board Certified Naturopathic Medical Doctor, there are a few issues regarding treatment of hypothyroidism. He believes patients are not prescribed the right type of thyroid medication and that even if they are prescribed the right type, they may not be taking enough of it.[i] Dr. Robinson recommends a natural thyroid supplement called Nature Throid, which includes T1, T2, T3 and T4 and in his experience it has been proven to work better, over the normally prescribed synthetic T4 hormone. He advocates for listening more closely to the patient and working with them instead of relying solely on what the blood panel says.[ii]

An alternative perspective comes from Marc Ryan, L.Ac., who is a practitioner of functional medicine and mainly treats those with Hashimoto's thyroiditis. He is of the opinion that some thyroid patients are prescribed too much of a thyroid hormone and even if it is a natural option, if the right conditions do not exist in the body for conversion then the medication will not work. Too much medication can cause an over abundance of the thyroxine (T4) hormone, which cannot convert and absorb into the cells properly and therefore he believes there are other natural options which can help with the conversion and absorption of this hormone.[iii]

Without going into more scientific, nerd stuff, outlined in chapter 4 are a few of his recommendations. Along with these we will discuss another effective strategy that can provide relief and supplement medications: essential oils. We will look at them in detail in the following chapters.

Chapter 3
The Fruit of the Earth
(or Aromatherapy: History
and Use)

The previous chapters, provided an overview of the thyroid gland and its function in the body, now, we will look at the history and use of essential oils. The word "aromatherapy" was not in use until 1937 when René Maurice Gattefossé, a french perfume chemist, wrote a book called *Aromathérapie*. He had an experience, in 1910, with lavender oil preventing gaseous, gangrenous sores from spreading on his skin after burns from an explosion in his laboratory. He reported that he poured lavender oil on his sores and they started healing the day after he administered the oil. This lead him to start working with the military to help heal soldiers with gangrene, using essential oils instead of antiseptics. Gattefossé is credited as the grandfather of aromatherapy, especially in regards to its practice as a healing agent.

What are essential oils?

Essential oils are naturally occurring oils that are extracted from natural resources such as leaves, roots, bark, flowers etc. They are the essence or quintessence of these plant substances. These contain concentrated levels of natural, aromatic compounds that are full of goodness and very potent. These volatile aromatic compounds change from solid to gas at room temperature and evaporate quickly.

Have you ever wondered what is actually contained in the blue smoke or mist that is suspended in the Smoky Mountains of Tennessee? According to David Stewart, in his book, *The Chemistry of Essential Oils*, the smoke is not actually smoke or even fog, "It is a cloud of essential oil molecules emitted by the trees to blanket the forest and reduce evaporation to preserve moisture." Further research suggests that there are even more reasons for this so called smoke. The trees and plants use it to protect themselves through the production of hydrocarbons called terpenes. Viruses, fungi and bacteria cannot survive when terpenes are present. A-pinene (a monoterpene), which is a common terpene derived from most vegetation, is a natural insecticide. Furthermore, there are monoterpene's found in flowers that attract certain insects and repel others. God knew what He was doing when He created the Earth. What a thought!

The greatest thing about this is that God made these plants for human beings as well and we can be the beneficiaries of their amazing healing properties. As Mark Kohler, on The Oil Academy blog, points out, a-pinene is an acetylcholinesterase inhibitor, fancy for, it helps you remember things. He says, "…it can promote alertness and memory retention and is also known as a bronchodilator (an agent that causes dilation of the bronchial tubes by relaxing bronchial muscle) which is potentially helpful for asthmatics." These are some key factors to remember for those who suffer from thyroid imbalances that can lead to a foggy memory and possibly asthma.

Essential oils find their use in many industries including cosmetics, personal care products and the food industry. But one industry that extensively uses essential oils is the medical industry, even if only, widely, by a few select practitioners. Essential oils are known for their medicinal properties and provide, sometimes quick, relief from various ailments and their symptoms. Anything from joint to muscle issues to depression and anxiety, essential oils are and meant to provide relief and can act as a supplement or a compliment to medication.

There are more than 3000 varieties (enough to overwhelm anyone, especially if you're wanting quick relief!) of aromatic compounds that have been identified to date and are used in the preparation of medicines created to treat various ailments. There are many pure essential oils that are extracted from quality ingredients sourced from organic farms, wildcrafted or sourced from their indigenous origin. There are also many that have been adulterated and sold as pure even though they have been mixed with other ingredients that lower their quality and hinder their effect on healing. The aromatic compounds in unadulterated essential oils vary from plant to plant as their concentration ratio depends on season and geography.

Essential oils can be used to provide relief from thyroid issues such as hyperthyroidism and hypothyroidism. There are many oils that can be used to stimulate the gland and help it release sufficient levels of thyroxine, as well as block its release in the case of hyperactivity. These oils are used to supplement medication and can provide relief from various symptoms.

How do essential oils work?

Essential oils, unlike conventional medicines, are made from natural compounds that are easier for the body to break down. These compounds are easily absorbed into the skin much like topically applied medicines. In fact, when applied to the skin, especially to the bottom of the feet, an essential oil can be found in all the cells of the body within

20 minutes. Once inside, they begin work on the various symptoms and provide quick relief. When it comes to thyroid issues, applying essential oils externally can help in stimulating the gland as well as inducing calm and relaxation. There are many different techniques that can be employed to enhance the effect of essential oils on your body such as the application of heat, usage of tools, reflexology coupled with the use of essential oils and more. We will discuss these in detail in chapters to come.

Chapter 4
The Sweet Spot
(or 27 Essential Oils to Help
Heal Your Thyroid: and
how they can help)

*FDA disclaimer: "The statements in regard to the implementation of essential oils or aromatherapy for the treatment of thyroid dysfunction or any other disease have not been evaluated by the Food and Drug Administration. These guidelines are not intended to diagnose, treat, cure, or prevent disease. *

As mentioned earlier, there are over 3000 types of essential oils and each one has a different effect on the body. In this chapter we will discuss some oils that are good for balancing the body and aid in relieving hypo and hyperthyroidism. Admittedly, there is a place for conventional medicine. But, the premise of this book is the idea that if a person uses natural and unadulterated methods to heal, conventional medicine will more than likely not be necessary. As Kurt Schnaubelt, writes in his book, *The Healing Intelligence of Essential Oils: The Science of Advanced Aromatherapy*, "The easy availability of antibiotics leads to lax prevention!"[iv]

The Keys for Thyroid Hormone Balancing and Healing

In order for the thyroid to be in balance and for the healing process to begin, there are a few key factors to keep in mind. The best way to determine what is happening in your body is to have a blood test done through a functional doctor who will order the correct test for you; an example of a sufficient test is provided in chapter 8. If you do not have the means to do this, it does not mean you cannot begin an essential oil regimen. The main reason that you can start right away is that essential oils aid in balancing your bodily functions, especially your hormonal activity. Because of their balancing effect, essential oils are an efficient natural remedy and can be used to aid in the key factors for improving thyroid function. These key factors can overwhelmingly be applied to hypothyroidism, but some of them can be applied to both and they are as follows: gut health, liver function, stress/cortisol levels, increased free T3 levels. The rest of this chapter will focus on these 4 important factors which can be applied to generally healthy thyroid function. For each factor, we will discuss specific essential oils and how they can help in dealing with these factors.

(1) Healing your Gut

The gut (the gastrointestinal tract) is one of the most important parts of the human body and the gut flora, also known as gut microbiota, which includes trillions of microorganisms that are made up of 1000 or more separate species of bacteria, is arguably the most important factor in your health. Most ailments stem from a damaged gut or an imbalance in gut flora. Having a healthy gut will lead to the healing of many other problems in the body.

Thyroid hormones function in the gut as well and this is where close to 20% of T4 converts to T3. Therefore, gut balance is of prime significance. An imbalance of thyroid hormones can also contribute to what is known as a "leaky gut." Leaky gut is a condition developed from a separation of the mesh that makes up the intestinal lining; small holes are developed and therefore the contents of the intestines can leak into the rest of the body and into the bloodstream. This can have damaging effects and causes substantial imbalances in the body. If you have SIBO (Small Intestine Bacterial Overgrowth), yeast overgrowth, acid reflux or intestinal dysbiosis, these are all signs of an imbalance in the, gut and/or thyroid. Intestinal sulfatase is a key enzyme found in the gut and is pivotal in the conversion of T4 to T3. If there is too much T4 hormone in your gut, inflammation will occur, which in turn raises cortisol and therefore will reduce active T3 hormone. Gut function and thyroid function go hand in hand and if one is out of whack the other will be too. Therefore, it will be important to address both simultaneously in order to achieve the proper balance.

Testing will help to determine where your specific imbalance occurs and working with a nutritionist will help to determine the proper foods to include in your diet. You can get the balancing process started by using the following essential oils. They are powerful in helping to balance gut flora or the flow of the metabolism, they include, cumin, marjoram, lavender, neroli, peppermint and thyme. An explanation of peppermint is found under the section, "Best essential oils for hypothyroidism" and thyme can be found in the next section, "Healing your liver." The rest can be found below.

Cumin

Latin name: **Cuminum cyminum**

If you have a sluggish and slow digestive system, cumin oil will be your best friend. It is comparable to coriander (description in the section "Increasing T3 levels") in the way it assists in digestion and these two will compliment each other well in a blend. Cumin invigorates and can be especially constructive in boosting the heart and nervous system. Cumin will help the body to break down food and digest more efficiently through the production of bile and the liberation of digestive enzymes. It also aids in preventing fermentation in the intestines. Cumin seeds have similar health benefits to its essential oil, but most of these benefits come from the essential oil, which is more potent than the seeds.

Appropriate uses:

Use in very small amounts and beware that cumin is photosensitive for 12 hours, which means that it can cause the skin to burn when exposed to sun.

Alone:

Dilute 2 drops of cumin essential oil with about a quarter teaspoon or more of sesame oil and rub in a clockwise direction in the area of your abdomen to stimulate and balance your digestive tract. Use 1 drop in your favorite tea. Use caution with internal use and do not ingest without diluting.

Blended:

To energize and relieve fatigue, blend 5 drops cumin with 5 drops each of lemon and clove and add to 1 tablespoon of your favorite carrier oil (fractionated coconut oil, grapeseed oil, sweet almond oil, hazelnut oil, jojoba oil, or borage oil). Massage this blend on the back of your neck, shoulders and chest in the morning to help you awaken.

Marjoram

Latin name: **Origanum majorana**

Marjoram is an amply versatile oil with diverse assets. A main attribute of marjoram is its role in bolstering peristalsis, which is how waste is moved along in the intestines by an expanding and contracting action. Marjoram creates warmth in the body and inhibits stagnation of joints and muscles. The warmth of marjoram can also dilate the arteries to minimize distress on the heart. At the same time, it is a sedative and can curtail insomnia.

Appropriate uses:

Blended as a Mist spray:

In an amber bottle that has a sprayer lid, combine with 4 fluid ounces of filtered water 30 drops of marjoram oil, 40 drops orange oil, 30 drops of lavender oil and 20 drops of sandalwood oil, close lid and shake. This blend aids in calming anxiety or insomnia. Spritz over head several times or on pillow before bed. Spray into the air to add a refreshing scent to any room. This is safe for children and can be used to calm hyperactivity.

Blended for Massage:

To relieve constipation, blend 3 drops marjoram with 3 drops of rosemary, 2 drops of chamomile and add to 5 teaspoons of your favorite carrier oil (fractionated coconut oil, grapeseed oil, sweet almond oil, hazelnut oil, jojoba oil, or borage oil). Massage this blend in a clockwise direction in the area of your lower abdomen and your lower back for a few minutes every day or every other day in the morning to help stimulate a bowel movement.

Lavender

Latin name: **Lavandula angustifolia or officinale**

Lavender is the most widely used essential oil and it is a feat to describe the multiplicity of advantageous characteristics. It is well known as a calming, anti-anxiety and sleep promoting oil. With regard, specifically to healing the gut, lavender helps to balance the bacteria in the gut and promote beneficial bacteria while prohibiting bacterial overgrowth. Lavender can also benefit the gut by reducing inflammation. Lavender is a best friend to antioxidants and in 2 separate research studies, one in China and one in Romania, it has been found that after using or inhaling the oil for 7 days in a row for an hour a day, the body will react by generating the 3 most important and powerful antioxidants called glutathione (the importance of this enzyme will be discussed in the next section"Healing Your Liver"), catalase (which accelerates, or catalyzes, the rate at which hydrogen peroxide ($H2O2$) is decomposed into water ($H2O$) and oxygen (O)), and SOD (stands for superoxide dismutase, which is another enzyme and it is very important in maintaining glutathione).Glutathione, catalase, and SOD all work together to help the body fight oxidative stress.

Appropriate uses:
In some ways, lavender could be the only essential oil you use and you would still get the many benefits of most of the rest. Lavender is one of the safest oils for most people, but it is still advised to be cautious and to use diluted with a carrier oil and to test it on a small part of your skin to be certain that you don't have a reaction. It is possible to experience sensitization with any essential oil, including lavender. With repeated use a reaction could develop and you could become sensitive to any oil, so it is important to rotate the oils you use on your skin.

Alone:
Use a solution of half lavender and half filtered water in a spray bottle and spritz on your pillow before bedtime. The Romanian research found that using lavender oil in a diffuser can help in fighting cancer, it will aid in protection of cells, preventing damage that can cause cancer. Use 15 drops with 1 cup of epsom salt in the bathtub for a relaxing 20-minute soak right before bed.

Blended:

Lavender blends well with bitter orange and cumin. A safe way to take this blend internally is by blending them in enteric coated capsules. Fill a glass, amber dropper bottle with equal parts of each oil and then drop this blend into one half of the capsule. It is important to work with a healthcare expert/professional to determine correct dosages for you.

Neroli

Latin name: **Citrus aurantium var. Amara**
Neroli is an oil derived from orange tree flowers and its emotional benefits are well worth mentioning, especially its help with anxiety and stress, in which it has been shown, in control group studies, to reduce immensely. It also enhances the effectiveness and proper functioning of the endocrine system and it will help you get a great night's sleep. Neroli's role in the gut stems from its anti-anxiety and anti-spasmodic properties; it can help calm the intestinal muscles and aid in lessening diarrhea, especially when it's caused by nervousness.

Appropriate uses:
Make sure to blend neroli with a carrier oil like sweet almond or jojoba oil if applied directly to the skin. Inhalation of neroli has been shown in control group studies to significantly reduce stress and blood pressure as well as to improve symptoms and increase sexual desire in postmenopausal women.

Alone:
Put 2 to 3 drops in a diffuser before bed to induce a deeper sleep. Combine 20 to 40 drops with double the amount of jojoba oil in an amber bottle with a steel roller ball and roll on your lower abdomen to help relieve diarrhea.

Blended:
To de-stress and manage mood swings, make up a blend of equal parts neroli, lavender, marjoram and ylang ylang to

fill 10 or 15 mL amber bottle with an orifice reducer or dropper. Inhale this concoction every morning and carry it with you all day taking a deep whiff every few hours or whenever you feel anxious. A good way to keep the scent on you all day is to purchase or make a diffuser necklace or bracelet that is made with dried clay.

(2) Healing Your Liver

The liver is what breaks down rT3, therefore it needs to be working properly in order for this action to occur. D1 (D'iodinase) is present in the liver and is needed to convert T4 to T3. As Marc Ryan points out, if there is a selenium deficiency in your body this process will be hindered. It is important to look out for heavy metals as well, especially mercury, lead and cadmium. If your body is harboring heavy metals, your liver is not working correctly.

Each cell present in your body contains a molecule called, glutathione, which is made up of 3 different amino acids (which are the building blocks for protein), called glycine, cysteine and glutamine. You can take glutathione in supplement form, which is recommended by Marc Ryan or, better yet, it can be found in certain foods, namely, raw milk (not pasteurized) from grass-fed cows or other animals, raw eggs from pastured chickens, red meats and organs from grass-fed cows or other animals, curcumin (will enhance the metabolism of glutathione), non-denatured whey protein from grass-fed cows, with no sweeteners or anything added to it (make sure it is cold-processed because heat will damage the proteins). Ryan also introduces nutrients such as, B vitamins, magnesium, glycine and sulfur as important aspects of liver function. There are a few essential oils that are best for liver function, including rosemary, chamomile, peppermint, cypress, lemon, thyme and juniper. Some are described in the following section and others will be described in other sections as they can have multiple ways of healing.

Rosemary

Latin name: **Rosmarinus officinalis**

Patricia Davis, in her book *Aromatherapy: An A-Z*, retells a legend about Rosemary, saying, "Legend says that the flowers were once white, but that they turned blue after the Virgin Mary hung her cloak on a rosemary bush when the Holy Family stopped to rest on the flight into Egypt."[v] Rosemary is obviously a special herb! Rosemary is antiseptic and has also been used in religious ceremonies for thousands of years, not only by Israelites and Christians, but also by Egyptians for embalming the dead. It is also used as a natural preservative for meat and other foods. Bile is important to the liver and the entire digestive system. Rosemary can enhance the functioning of the gallbladder and promote the generation and movement of bile, it can also be used for clearing up jaundice. It should be used in very small doses. Rosemary can relieve nausea and vomiting by inhibiting the neurotransmitter acetylcholine and can also help to detoxify and eliminate waste from the liver and digestive system. The warming effect of rosemary gets the circulation moving and opens up the blood vessels, helping in the healing process. In a study from Japan, rosemary and lavender were both found to reduce cortisol levels after inhaling their aroma for 5 minutes. Rosemary is also good for thickening and growing of hair and for chelating iron.

Appropriate uses:

Use rosemary in very small amounts and it should be avoided if your blood pressure is high. It is best not use if you are pregnant, nursing or trying to conceive or if you have a seizure disorder or epilepsy.

Alone:

For the purpose of improving bile flow and the performance of the gallbladder (which stores bile and secretes it in order to digest fat), combine 3 drops of rosemary oil with _ cup of grapeseed oil or fractionated coconut oil and apply to skin, twice a day, in the area of the gallbladder, located below the liver and ribs on the right side of the body.

Blended:

To energize your digestion, try this bath remedy. First mix together 3 drops rosemary, 2 drops chamomile, 4 drops lemongrass, 1 drop clary sage, 3 drops coriander, 1 tablespoon carrier oil of your choice (jojoba is good for a bath) and 1 tablespoon of milk, which is optional (it helps the oils to absorb into the water). Fill the bath with warm water and add a cup of epsom salt (optional, for added stress relief and especially effective right before bed). And the then add the mixture of oils and soak for at least 20 minutes.

Chamomile

Latin names: Eriocephalus punctulatus (Cape), Matricaria recutita or Chamaemelum matricaria (German), Tanacetum annuum (Morracan), Anthemis nobilis or Chamaemelum nobile (Roman)

Chamomile has a vast amount of different uses and has both physical and emotional benefits. There is a large amount of variations of chamomile, German chamomile is a variety that is often referenced, but they all have similar effects. Chamomile has, mainly calming and anti-inflammatory effects and therefore it can pacify anxiety or panic as well as reduce the inflammation that could be causing the anxiety. It can also be used as a treatment for insomnia, much like lavender. The German chamomile variety can be instrumental in increasing liver function by promoting bile secretion and detoxification and it is gentler than rosemary. Anodyne or pain reducing components are found in Roman chamomile. It is antispasmodic and therefore helps to relax and soothe the gut to promote better digestion and movement of food through the system.

Appropriate uses:

Chamomile has been reported to be a mild and safe oil with no side effects. It is advised to still use caution and do a patch test to be sure that you do not have a reaction.

Alone:

Apply 2 to 4 drops and rub in a clockwise direction on the abdominal area. Administer chamomile, especially to help with morning elimination and digestion in general, which will help to repair a leaky gut.

Blended:

For a liver detox, use a blend of 3 drops German chamomile, 4 drops cypress, 4 drops juniper, 5 drops geranium, 5 drops rosemary, 6 drops ginger. Use a 1 oz amber dropper bottle to contain the oils and fill to the top with sweet almond oil or a carrier oil of your choice. Apply this blend to the liver, abdomen and lower back area using approximately a dropperful. Or use the same blend, undiluted, dropped onto a cottonball and inhale every few minutes in the morning as you are getting ready or for five minutes at night, right before bed. The oils will absorb into your bloodstream quicker through the inhalation method and will absorb gradually throughout the day using the application method.

Cypress

Latin name: **Cupressus sempervirens**

Cypress is an aid in decongesting the liver and lowering cholesterol levels, according to a study that took place in 2007, in Cairo. It contains antioxidants that help to eliminate toxins. It will also help to inhale cypress in the case of an asthma attack, as it is an antispasmodic. Your menstrual cycle will benefit from cypress, which it will help to regulate and balance your hormonal cycle.

Appropriate uses:
Do not ingest cypress oil. Do not use while pregnant, it is not known whether it is safe to use on children. Always use a carrier oil when applying to skin.

Alone:
To calm anxiety and eliminate toxins, add 5 to 7 drops of cypress oil to a diffuser nearby and keep it going for no more than an hour at a time. Or add the same amount to a cotton ball and inhale every few minutes an hour before bedtime.

Blended:
Make a natural face wash for deep cleansing and detoxification, acne prevention and age/sun spot reduction. Mix together in a glass jar, 1 cup fractionated coconut oil, 1 tbsp baking soda, 5 drops each of lavender, frankincense and lemon and 1 to 3 drops of cypress and store in a dark, cool place. Massage onto face for 2 minutes every morning and evening. If you do not want to worry about sun exposure, replace lemon with lemongrass.

Lemon

Latin name: **Citrus limonum**
Lemon oil has been reported to prevent stagnation in the liver since 1964 when Jean Valnet wrote about it. Lemon and orange are extremely powerful aids to liver detoxification. Carcinogens cannot remain in the vicinity of citrus oils because of the limonene substance contained in them. This substance also stops the reproduction of tumor cells. Kurt Schnaubelt promotes the ingestion of lemon oil for liver detoxification by adding 1 or 3 drops to water and stirring before drinking. This should only be done with 3 or less drops of organic lemon oil, without pesticides. In a study coming out of India, the compound contained in lemon oil called hesperidin was reported to block lipopolysaccharide (LPS)-induced endotoxicity in rats. LPS

causes the secretion of cytokines from cells, which can increase inflammation. Hesperidin has been shown to reduce inflammation and oxidative stress.

Appropriate uses:

Keep in mind that when topically applying lemon oil it will be photosensitive for 12 hours, which means that it can cause the skin to burn when exposed to the sun. Remember to patch test.

Alone:

For a liver detox, mix together 1/8 tsp organic, raw honey and 1/4 tsp organic, raw coconut oil, add one drop of lemon oil and consume orally.

Blended:

For better sleep and relaxation, in a 3 or 4 oz amber dropper bottle, combine 6 drops lemon, 8 drops chamomile, 10 drops lavender oil and 2 oz or 4 tbsp sweet almond oil and shake to blend. Rub on neck chest and temples one hour before bed or use a dropperful in a espom salt bath, soaking for 20 minutes.

Thyme

Latin name: **Thymus vulgaris**

Thyme cannot only preserve meat from going bad, mostly in the plant form, but can also protect your immune system from pathogens and jump start digestion, which is especially helpful for a metabolism that is slowed down from hypothyroidism. Thyme acts in the defense of the body to protect it from foreign invaders because it helps the body to generate white corpuscles, which are blood cells that surround and ingest fungi and bacteria. If you suffer from fatigue and lethargy, thyme will help to stimulate you and wake you up, but at the same time it is balancing because it will help you to sleep when you suffer from insomnia. It is also a brain stimulant. The linalool in thyme can cause regeneration and detoxification in the liver. Skin healing and regeneration is another wonderful property of thyme.

Appropriate uses:

Thyme oil is mostly safe when used in small amounts. There is a possibility of an allergic reaction and you should take heed if you are allergic to oregano or any other member of the Lamiaceae species because it is likely that you are allergic to thyme as well. Skin application is usually safe, but should be tested for irritation. Thyme can slow down the development of blood clots, so be cautious and do not use thyme if you have a blood disease or are going into surgery within a couple weeks. Use caution if pregnant.

Alone:

To help with circulation diffuse 2-3 drops of thyme essential oil daily. If it doesn't cause irritation, it is safe to use directly on the skin to heal scars caused by acne.

Blended:

To decongest the liver use a blend of 3 drops thyme, 3 drops cypress and 3 drops lemon with 1 TBSP of fractionated coconut oil and rub over the liver, located below the ribs on the right side, before you go to bed at night.

(3) Reducing Stress/Lowering cortisol levels

It is inevitable that you have a stress problem, especially if you have thyroid problems. Most people who have an ailment and visit the doctor are there because of stress even though they may not know it. In order to reduce stress, these 3 things are a requirement; lower cortisol levels, improve adrenal function and get more and better sleep.

I know, I know, everyone always says "get more sleep." As if you don't know that it's good to get more sleep. But, what if you CAN'T sleep?? This is the problem, and stress can be a part of the reason. Reducing stress can help you to get the deep and restful sleep you need and there are many essential oils described in this book which have an added benefit of reducing stress and inducing sleep. Some include, lavender (of course), ylang ylang, marjoram, chamomile, thyme and lemongrass.

Marc Ryan warns to be wary of prednisone and other corticosteroids as they can block D1 and increase D3 which can be detrimental in the conversion of T4 to T3. Your levels of dehydroepiandrosterone (or DHEA) and cortisol have to be in check. Dr. David Jockers is a Maximized Living doctor, corrective care chiropractor, nutritionist, exercise physiologist, and certified strength & conditioning specialist and he offers many insights into the DHEA hormone, which is vital in optimal adrenal function. Increased production of DHEA is necessary for many functions in the body.[vi] One of his suggestions is to use aromatherapy, he says, "The aromatherapy of essential oils can help to reduce stress and improve neurotransmitter function. Additionally, they have a positive effect on anti-aging hormone production. Some of the best for this include lavender, ylang-ylang, sandalwood and peppermint."

You must gain the ability to manage your stress by getting enough sleep, controlled relaxation through breathing and stretching exercises, spending time outdoors, prayer, massage and aromatherapy. Other ways to balance your adrenal function are to take an adrenal supplement, reduce or completely eliminate caffeine, consume more salt (no table salt, but unrefined and raw: sea salt, pink Himalayan salt, Celtic grey salt or Real salt) and take care of any nutrient deficiencies in your body.

Many essential oils can be used to reduce stress and the strain on the adrenals, some of those are Chamomile, Clary Sage, Jasmine, Lavender, Marjoram, Neroli, Rose, Rosewood, Vetivert, Geranium, Rosemary, Black Pepper,

Peppermint and Thyme. Below are two oils that are not mentioned in other sections of this chapter.

Geranium

Latin name: **Pelargonium graveolens**

Geranium oil is actually derived from steam distilling the leaves and stem of the plant and not the petals of the flower. Geranium has antiseptic and antidepressant elements within it. Geranium is very important in stimulating the adrenal cortex, the outside part of the adrenal gland that produces hormones and synthesizes corticosteroid and androgen hormones. The job of these hormones is to create balance in the hormones that other organs secreted. Detoxification of the liver and kidneys is another benefit. Quercetin is an important flavonoid found in geranium, which, mostly notably, has been found to lessen the spread of cancer cells.

Appropriate uses:

Be sure to use geranium earlier in the day and in small amounts because it can tend to be over stimulating and agitating if over used.

Alone:

For adrenal health, geranium can be applied directly to the adrenal glands, located directly under the ribs in the middle of the back. It is important to use a carrier oil to dilute the oil, especially if you have sensitive skin. Use 1-2 drops per tsp of carrier oil. It can also be applied to the soles of the feet to take advantage of the absorption from the largest pores in the body, especially if digestion is difficult.

Blended:

To relieve adrenal fatigue, transfer this blend into a 4oz amber bottle; ½ tsp clove, 1 tsp geranium, 1 tsp chamomile, 2 tsp lemongrass and 2 tsp frankincense. When applying to the skin combine 5-6 drops of this solution with sweet almond oil or a carrier oil of your choice. This can also be used in a bath and as soak for the feet. An alternative method that requires a larger batch, involves using a cotton cloth and heating one cup of carrier oil and adding 30 drops of your adrenal fatigue blend above. Dip the cloth in the warm mix and apply to the adrenals, just above the kidneys.

Black Pepper

Latin name: **Piper nigrum**

Black pepper is a highly prized spice. The essential oil is especially good for the gut. It can strengthen the adrenals as well. Black pepper oil is a stimulant, but an antispasmodic as well, therefore it can create balance in the digestive system. It can also stimulate the secretion of hydrochloric acid in the stomach, which helps in more effective digestion. This oil can also lead to better sexual function and hormone balancing, so that's always good.

<u>Appropriate uses:</u>

It would be a mistake to use too much of this oil, but in small quantities it can be very energizing to a sluggish thyroid or slow body. It is warming when applied to the skin, so it is essential to do a patch test. Do not use before bed.

Alone:

Black pepper can be taken orally as long as you have the purest and best possible product you can find and use a 1:1 dilution with a carrier oil, olive oil is a suggestion. One to two drops can be added to a soup, broth or smoothie to relieve diarrhea or constipation.

Blended:

To refresh and energize, combine 1 drop black pepper, 1 drop cinnamon, 2 drops cypress and 3 drops lemon and diffuse. Enjoy this wonderful scent!

(4) Increasing Free T3 levels

There are 5 main actions that need to happen in order for free T3 levels to be increased. These 5 actions are to reduce rT3, improve conversion of T4 to T3, increase nutrient absorption, lower overall inflammation and reverse leptin and insulin resistance.

Zinc and Selenium are key nutrients in helping to reduce inflammation. Zinc also helps to produce thyroid stimulating hormone, along with magnesium and vitamins B-12. Dietary fat in the form of healthy oils, like coconut or olive oil, raw cheese, nuts or meat, is required in order for your body to efficiently absorb vitamins and nutrients from food that you eat or supplements that you take. Another way to help with nutrients is to eat nutrient dense foods like, organ meats (it's always good to get the worst one out of the way first!), green leafy vegetables, root vegetables and probiotic rich foods like kombucha or fermented vegetables (which is the topic of my second book in this series, called *Fermentation and Thyroid Health*). Regarding essential oils, Robert Tisserand, a renowned aromatherapist, says, "There is no evidence showing that essential oil constituents can enhance the absorption of nutrients through cell walls, though it is a feasible concept."[vii] In this article, Tisserand also addresses a myth that has been perpetrated that essential oils help with oxygenation in the body. He debunks and corrects this myth saying that what essential oils have been shown to do is reduce oxidative stress, which is cell damage that happens because of oxygen.

Ryan once again emphasizes the power of glutathione, which also has a benefit of reducing inflammation in the body. Inflammation greatly hinders the conversion of T4 to T3 and can cause many other problems in the body, including the overproduction of cortisol.

Increased levels of leptin and/or insulin in your body also promote the increase of reverse T3, therefore it is necessary to reverse leptin and insulin resistance so that rT3 levels will be lowered. These two work together and can effect each other.[viii]

There are at least two ways aromatherapy can help with increasing free T3 levels, one is to improve insulin sensitivity and balance blood sugar. The use of cinnamon oil and coriander oil have been shown to help with this process.[ix] The other is to lower inflammation in the body. The best essential oils to use to reduce inflammation are ginger, peppermint, lavender and chamomile. The properties of these oils are outlined below or in other sections of this chapter.

Cinnamon

Latin names: **Cinnamomum verum (bark), Cinnamomum zeylanicum (leaf)**

Cinnamon is a member of the Lauraceae botanical family and has a large list of health benefitting qualities.

Cinnamon oil can either come from the bark or the leaf. The oil from bark is much more irritant than the oil from the leaf, therefore it is only advised to use the oil from the leaf on the skin in very small amounts as it can still be agitating to the skin, especially if you are prone to this. Although, there are differing thoughts in the aromatherapy world on cinnamon bark and leaf oil and on whether it should be ingested or not. It is advisable to use caution and common sense when determining whether this oil will be right for you. It is a very powerful oil and has antibacterial and antispasmodic qualities and could bring strong benefits for some. It can aid in the reduction of inflammation, as well as speed up circulation and fight depression.

Cinnamon and its oil have been found in at least one study to promote the inhibition of insulin resistance. It also aids the pancreas in balancing blood sugar[x] and boosts the immune system, among many other benefits.

Appropriate uses:

Although it is considered safe to ingest by the FDA, it is important, if ingested, that it be the best and most-pure and an organic option.

Alone:

Cinnamon oil administered in suppository form is an idea for a very safe option that will produce benefits. If diffused, the oil from the bark will produce the aroma that is common for cinnamon, Christmas will be in the air! The leaf is a more woodsy aroma. It will help keep the flu away!

Blended:

To stimulate your scalp, if you are experiencing hair loss, try this scalp massage recipe. Gradually increase the amount of essential oil used to test for irritation. Slight tingling is the goal and nothing more. Warm 2 TBS of raw and unrefined extra virgin coconut oil and combine with 3 drops lemon oil, 2 drops peppermint oil and 1 to 5 drops cinnamon oil. Massage into scalp for a few minutes before showering.

Coriander

Latin name: **Coriandrum savitum**

Both coriander essential oil, derived from the seeds used to produce cilantro, and coriander seeds have many digestive and liver healing benefits. Coriander can regulate and balance the blood sugar levels in the liver and therefore improve insulin sensitivity, similar to cinnamon. It can also help relieve bloating and gas by encouraging digestion. Boosted energy and reduced pain are additional "side effects" of coriander.

Appropriate uses:

Coriander oil is generally not toxic or irritating when not taken in excess. Use caution and work with your physician if using internally. Skin and intestinal complications could develop if used in excessive amounts.

Alone:
Take an enteric coated capsule, including 8-10 drops of coriander oil, daily if approved by your healthcare professional.
Blended:
Diffuse this blend of 2 drops of coriander and 1 drop each of cinnamon and ginger. For an aid in improving digestion make this blend to massage onto the stomach in a clockwise direction around the belly button. Using a 2 oz amber bottle, combine 3 drops each of coriander and peppermint, 6 drops ginger and 8 drops lemongrass. This blend will truly awaken your senses!

Ginger

Latin name: **Zingiber officinale**
Ginger is a very powerful, healing root and can be used in a variety of ways. Ginger in the form of the essential oil is more robust than the raw root because it has a higher content of gingerol, which is what contains the healing characteristics. Ginger is well known for treating nausea and it is very effective in alleviating it. Among other things, it is very anti-inflammatory, which is attributed to one of its components called zingibain. A study on mice showed that when mice were administered ginger oil for a month, they had increased enzyme levels and lowered inflammation. Increased enzyme levels will also help your body to absorb more nutrients! Many studies have indicated that ginger should be utilized routinely.

Appropriate uses:
There are few occurrences of negative side effects from using ginger oil, at most, if used in very high amounts, it can cause slight heartburn, mouth irritation or diarrhea. If you are using blood thinner, diabetes or high blood pressure medication, it can be risky to use ginger oil and it is best not to use it in these cases.

Alone:
Homemade ginger oil infusion: After rinsing and letting 1 cup of fresh ginger dry for around 3 hours, chop and shred the ginger with a cheese grater, put into a stoneware, ceramic or tempered glass bowl and add 1 ½ cups extra virgin olive oil. Put in oven at 150° F for two hours or more. Strain with an unbleached cheese cloth and put into amber glass bottles. Good for up to 6 months. Use small amounts (1-2 drops) in cooking, diffuse and use as a massage (2-3 drops) on the abdomen.
Blended:
For a room spritz, use a 4 oz spray bottle and add 3 drops ginger oil and 5 drops orange oil and fill with filtered water. Use the same amounts of both oils in a diffuser.

Best Essential Oils for Hypothyroidism

Hypothyroidism is a condition where the thyroid gland does not secrete enough thyroxine in the body. This can lead to complications such as Hashimoto's disease. Although medicines are administered to treat hypothyroidism, there are some essential oils that can provide relief from its symptoms and they are as follows.

Peppermint

Latin name: **Mentha piperita**
Peppermint or spearmint greatly helps in reducing fatigue thereby making it one of the most recommended essential oils to treat hypothyroidism. These aid in the secretion of thyroid hormones. It lends the body strength and support in order to fix the weakness brought about by the condition. Peppermint stills inflammation and also stimulates the body, including the immune system and can ease stomach

discomfort. It has been shown to be very effective in treating Irritable Bowel Syndrome (see treatment below). It can also produce a clearer mind and elevate the mood if one struggles with depression.

Appropriate uses:
Do not apply on or near the face infants or children. There is some anecdotal evidence reporting that peppermint can lower milk supply when breastfeeding. Peppermint can be a skin irritant and should never be used "neat" without a carrier oil. It is not recommended to take orally in water.

Alone:
Peppermint can be put into enteric coated capsules and taken orally or can be purchased over the counter to treat IBS.

Blended:
Every morning, use a 2 oz amber glass roller bottle filled with 3 drops each of peppermint, geranium, lemongrass and frankincense combined with rosehip or fractionated coconut oil. Roll onto the base of your neck where your thyroid is located and onto your lower back where your adrenals are located, below the ribs.

Clary sage

Latin name: **Salvia sclarea**
Clary sage is a go-to essential oil for all who wish to put an end to brain fogginess. It helps in clearing out stress, increasing brain function and is an aid in the balancing of hormones. There have been a myriad of studies done on clary sage, especially pertaining to hormones. Clary sage has been shown in this research study to have reduced the levels of cortisol in the bodies of depression prone women by 36% after inhalation.[xi] It was also found to be anti-depressant and can also relax symptoms of PCOS and menstrual pain. Clary sage contains esters which cause

regulation in the pituitary gland, therefore having a positive effect on the entire endocrine system.

Appropriate uses:

There are not many contraindications that come with clary sage oil. It is recommended to avoid using during the first 3 months of pregnancy, just as a caution, especially if you have a history of miscarriages. Though there is no evidence or research that suggests that it has caused miscarriage, some have expressed worry due to it being an emmenagogue oil, meaning it can causing heavy bleeding during the menstrual cycle.

Alone:

If you do not have a diffuser, boil some water and add 3 drops of clary sage oil and take deep, long breathes in to reduce stress at the close of the day.

Blended:

When combined with ylang ylang oil, clary sage can lift libido due to its aphrodisiac effects, plus it causes a wonderful aroma. Diffuse a couple drops of each in the bedroom!

Orange

Latin name: **Citrus sinensis**

The orange peel is what produces orange oil. The main constituent in orange oil is limonene, which is a monoterpene that has been shown to prevent the growth of tumors in rats and rodents.[xii] Orange has been known to control stress, decrease anxiety and enhance thyroid function. Among many other desirable benefits, it helps to reduce oxidative stress, is anti-inflammatory and anti-cancer. It is also one of the least expensive oils to buy.

Appropriate uses:

Due to orange being a citrus oil, it can be photosensitive, so it is best to stay out of direct sunlight for at least 12 hours if using orange oil on the skin. Orange oil can be used on the skin, but it is important to do a patch test and start out with a very small amount so that a reaction does not occur.

Alone:

For a facial treatment to reduce wrinkles and acne: in a glass jar, combine 20 drops orange oil, 1 tbsp raw coconut oil, 3 tbsp raw honey, 1 tbsp apple cider vinegar and 2 capsules live probiotics and blend with a hand blender. Recipe courtesy of www.draxe.com.

Blended:

Orange, clove and peppermint blend well together. Add 3 drops of each to a diffuser and enjoy the delicious aroma. Orange is also very powerful is used with frankincense or cinnamon to reduce wrinkles because is activates the production of collagen.

Clove

Latin name: **Syzygium aromaticum**

Clove oil is a very powerful oil to use for balancing the endocrine system. Clove has an extremely high anti-oxidant capacity, it's ORAC score is over 1,000,000. It is also extremely high in phenols which detoxify receptor sites in cells, which is required for cells to communicate and keep the body healthy. Clove can also be used to treat neurological difficulties which may arise due to hypothyroidism, like depression and anxiety, it helps decrease mental fatigue and stress. Also, it can get rid of bad breath and generally good for oral health, which is always good. Eugenol makes of 90 percent of clove oil and this is the component that gives it most of its healing properties.

Appropriate uses:

Clove can cause a stinging sensation when applied to the skin. Clove bud oil is the gentler than clove leaf or stem oil (which are not used in aromatherapy because of their very high potency). Can slow the blood clotting process because of how much eugenol it contains. It is recommended not to use, consistently, longer than 2 weeks.

Alone:
Add 3 to 5 drops to your bath water to treat digestive issues. It is very effective in cleaning the air and keeping away sickness if diffused in the home as well.

Blended:
For thyroid support make this blend to roll on your feet before bed: In a 10 mL amber bottle, combine, 20 drops each of clove, frankincense, myrrh, marjoram and lemongrass and fill to the top with fractionated coconut oil.

Best Essential Oils for Hyperthyroidism

Lemon balm

Latin name: **Melissa officinalis**
Lemon balm or Melissa oil is generally prescribed for those who suffer from hyperthyroidism. Lemon balm helps in curbing anxiety and providing relief from some of the symptoms associated with thyroid dysfunction due to an overactive thyroid. Research on lemon balm has found that if it encounters any sugar, it is able to devour it.[xiii] Lemon balm has also been shown to lower the thyroid stimulating hormone by inhibiting the thyroid-stimulating immunoglobulin G (Graves' IgG), which is similar to TSH, from binding to the TSH receptor.[xiv]

Appropriate uses:
Although it is a very mild oil, lemon balm should not be used by those taking thyroid medication, such as thyroxine, as it has been shown to block the action of this medication. Also, it is thought that it should not be used for those with

hypothyroidism, even though there are differing views on this. It can also act as a sleep inducer or sedative. Use caution when buying lemon balm as it has been adulterated with other oils in the past, be sure that it is pure lemon balm.

Alone:
Apply 1 to 2 drops on the wrists, the back of the neck or behind the ears. Add 5 drops to a small spray bottle and fill with water to use as a spritzer on your face. Add a couple drops to your favorite herbal tea to help with digestion.

Blended:
Blend lemon balm in a diffuser with geranium, lavender and orange or lemon oil, 2 or 3 drops each.

Jasmine

Latin name: **Jasminum officinale**

Jasmine essential oil is extremely soothing and provides relief from stress and anxiety. This helps in calming down the pituitary gland, and in turn, the thyroid. It is also a powerful antidepressant and aids in the secretion of serotonin. It helps to ease sleep disturbances and decrease insomnia. Jasmine has also been known to balance reproductive hormones and regulate the menstrual cycle.

Appropriate uses:
Do not use while pregnant, until labor and delivery due to emmenagogue properties. If used in very high quantities, it may cause sedation.

Alone:
Diffuse during bedtime routine or put a few drops on pillow before bed.

Blended:
For a wonderful and calming perfume, combine 30 drops jasmine oil with 5 drops each of sandalwood, lavender, orange and neroli, plus 2 TBS vodka. Put mixture in small perfume or spray bottle and fill with water.

Ylang Ylang

Latin name: **Cananga odorata var. Genuana**

One of my personal favorites, Ylang ylang is effective in providing relief from symptoms associated with hyperthyroidism. It is regarded as a sedative since it can induce drowsiness and make a person sleepy. It also normalizes heartbeat and is effective in controlling high blood pressure. It almost instantly calms me and lifts my mood with just one sniff.

Appropriate uses:

The floral aroma of ylang ylang is not for everyone and may be considered potent or pungent and could bring on a headache if too much is used.

Alone:

Rub on wrists and base of neck when diluted with fractionated coconut oil or almond oil.

Blended:

Ylang-ylang combined with clary sage is a divine aroma that will calm your nerves and help you to relax. Use 3 to 5 drops of each in a diffuser This will help normalize your heartbeat and lower cortisol. It is especially useful before bed.

Juniper

Latin name: **Juniperus communis**

The main components of juniper berries are flavonoids and polyphenols, which are powerful in keeping bacteria and infections at bay. Juniper berry oil is effective in detoxifying the body and used to provide relief from hyperthyroidism. It has a calming effect on a person and relieves stress and anxiety and can induce relaxation. Digestive enzymes have been shown to be activated in the presence of juniper oil, which helps to properly digest proteins and assimilate nutrients, it can also cleanse the liver.

Appropriate uses:
When applying to skin, juniper should be diluted in a 1:1 ratio with a carrier oil.

Alone:
Juniper oil can be digested as long as it is a very high quality oil and diluted. Mix 1 to 2 drops in water, juice or your favorite smoothie.

Blended:
Combine 20 or so drops each of juniper, lavender and chamomile in a small spray bottle with water. Spritz on pillows before bed to induce sleep or use as an air freshener.

Best Essential Oils for Both

Frankincense

Latin name: **Boswellia carterii or serrata or frareana**
Frankincense is an all around amazing essential oil, it has many powerful properties and has been used for thousands of years. It can be used to decrease the levels of stress in the body. It has also been known to decrease inflammation, decrease anxiety, help with reducing symptoms of asthma, aid in fighting cancer, improve immunity, improve skin conditions. Frankincense is used to provide relief from several symptoms associated with hypothyroidism. It deals with the weakness and constipation associated with the condition and also relieves digestive issues. It works like a digestive enzyme and breaks down food at a faster pace thereby preventing indigestion, bloating, flatulence and the like. Frankincense is also used to balance out the hormonal level and curb stress.

Appropriate uses:

Frankincense in the form of boswellia serrata can cause problems with Warfarin, a blood clotting medication and can thin the blood. In rare cases, has contributed to minor skin irritation and upset stomach.

Alone:

Combine 2 drops of frankincense with a tablespoon of raw honey to help with the digestive difficulties mentioned above. Frankincense can also be mixed with jojoba oil and rubbed on the skin to reduce wrinkles, use 6 drops of frankincense to one ounce of jojoba oil.

Blended:

For an anti aging serum combine 2 drops each of frankincense, lavender, geranium, jasmine, sandalwood and 1 ounce of jojoba or apricot kernel oil in an amber glass dropper bottle and use 3 drops on face before moisturizing.

Myrrh

Latin name: **Commiphora myrrha**

Myrrh is a highly beneficial oil. It has been used for healing since ancient times, it was a staple for soldiers in ancient Greece who carried it with them at all times and it can be used for a variety of purposes. It is made by steam distilling the resin of the commiphora myrrha tree and is "cousins" with Frankincense. Myrrh is especially helpful to the digestive tract and to rebalancing the systems of the body, including the immune system, the endocrine system (the system that includes the thyroid), nervous system and psychological system (therefore, it can help with emotions as well) and it has a very strong effect on all of these systems. It is also a pain killer and can drain toxins from the body.

Appropriate uses:

If you are diabetic use caution and consult your doctor before using myrrh, as it has been shown in some studies done on animals that myrrh can have hypoglycemic reactions. It can also cause problems with Warfarin, a blood clotting medication.

Alone:
Dilute 2 drops of myrrh essential oil with about a quarter teaspoon or more of jojoba oil and rub at the base of the neck in the area of your thyroid to stimulate and balance your hormones.

Blended:
For relaxation diffuse 1 to 2 drops each of myrrh, frankincense, sandalwood and orange. To use this blend often combine equal amounts of all oils in a 2 mL amber bottle (you can double the amount of the orange if it is to your liking).

Myrtle

Latin name: **Myrtus communis**

Myrtle is regarded as one of the best essential oils to use for thyroid issues, as it establishes a balance, as it is an adaptogen. If you suffer from hypothyroidism, then it stimulates the thyroid to release an adequate amount into the body. If you suffer from hyperthyroidism, then it curbs the release of thyroxine. Either way, you stand to benefit greatly from the use of this essential oil.

Appropriate uses:
Myrtle is mostly safe, but always dilute and use caution. Do not use on pets. It is safe to use with food, but 6 years and under should not ingest.

Alone:
Add a few drops of myrtle to a warm bath. Or combine a few drops in a bowl of warm water and soak a washcloth to use on the face or chest before bed.

Blended:
Combine 15 drops each of myrtle, frankincense and myrrh with 44 drops of sweet almond oil in an amber roller bottle and role directly over the thyroid area.

Lemongrass

Latin name: **Cymbopogon flexuosus**

Lemongrass is a grass that is native to India. If you suffer from insomnia or any type of restlessness due to either an underactive (a.k.a. active at the wrong times) or overactive thyroid or anything else, lemongrass will help to calm your mind and nerves down because of its sedative attributes. Yet, Lemongrass is also energizing with a fresh and invigorating aroma. It has also been used in alleviating headaches. 75% to 85% of lemongrass oil contains the compound called citral. Citral is a powerful detoxifier and can, reportedly, activate the important enzyme called glutathione-S-transferase (discussed in the section "Healing Your Liver"). Citral also has other powerful benefits, including skin cancer prevention.

Appropriate uses:

Use in small amounts and diluted with carrier oil, can cause irritation or burning if not diluted. The scent is very strong. Do not use with diabetes drugs or hypertensive medications.

Alone:

During your morning shower, use a few drops of lemongrass to create an envigorating and energizing spa experience, a perfect start to the day.

Blended:

In a 15 mL amber bottle combine 4 drops each of lemongrass, ylang ylang, orange and sandalwood and fill with grapeseed oil for an aphrodisiacal massage.

Sandalwood

Latin name: **Santalum spicatum (Australian), Santalum album (Indian)**

Sandalwood oil, used in Ayurvedic preparations, provides substantial relief from hyperthyroidism. It has a sedative and antispasmodic reaction and it is prescribed to those who suffer from hypertension, as it can effectively calm a person down. Sandalwood can also help regulate and lower testosterone levels in both men and women, which can help with hypothyroid problems.

Appropriate uses:

Always mix with carrier oil. There are no other known contraindications in association with sandalwood oil.

Alone:

Due to its manly and woodsy scent it is recommended to use in a homemade deodorant or cologne, for men.

Blended:

To reduce the appearance of stretch marks make this formula: 1 cup coconut oil, ¼ cup cocoa butter, 1/8 cup shea butter, 1/8 cup almond oil, 15 drops each of sandalwood, neroli and orange oils. In a double boiler, melt and blend coconut oil, cocoa butter, shea butter and almond oil. Then add essential oils after letting it cool slightly. Store in a sterile container. Recipe courtesy of www.essentialoilsanctuary.com

Essential oils are the best at helping with 5 elements related to the above Key factors in thyroid health, which are: gut health, stress reduction, liver detoxification, lowered inflammation and improved sleep. They will also help with generally balancing your bodily processes and they are powerful anti-oxidants as well. Essentials oils are pleasant and powerful and can be used as supplements to help you in different aspects of thyroid balance.

Note: Essential oils are not a magic formula or cure all. They are very powerful and healing oils from plant sources made by God. But, without a diet tailored to your specific symptoms and proper exercise, your results and the amount of relief you experience will be very limited. The solutions provided in this book are intended for long-term implementation. Do not expect long lasting results without regular, daily usage. Please consult your licensed healthcare professional about your specific symptoms or for testing and a healthcare regimen.

Are you receiving benefit from this book? Please leave a review!

Chapter 5
I Inhaled!
(or Aromatherapy
Methods: Topical, Oral,
Inhalation and Reflexology)

In the previous chapter, we looked at the different types of essential oils that can be used to treat hypo and hyperthyroidism. Let us now look at how these oils can be used.

Methods to Make Your Own Essential Oils

If you do not trust the oils you get in stores or you do not want to pay as much, then you can make some of your own. Although it can seem daunting, it is quite simple to extract essential oils. Here are some simple methods to do so.

1. Steam distiller method

The steam distiller method will require the purchase of a steam distiller starting at around $200. Therefore, it will not be cost effective on the front end, but if you buy a quality distiller it will last you for years to come. The model you purchase will have detailed instructions on how to extract the oils from the plant and you will understand why a lot of essential oils are higher priced

2. Pressure cooker method

Ingredients:
#1: leaves, stems and flowers of the plant you wish to extract oil from (rose, jasmine, lavender, bay leaves, orange peels etc.) Ensure they are fresh and personally collected to ensure quality
#2: 1 pressure cooker
#3: good quality sealant
#4: heat resistant rubber tube
#5: tub of cold water
#6: beaker
#7: sterilized glass jars

Method:
Step 1: Use the sealant to cover the open valve of the cooker.
Step 2: Attach the rubber pipe to the steam valve and use the sealant to secure it.
Step 3: Place the cooker on a stove and add in the raw ingredients after washing them thoroughly.
Step 4: Add enough water to cover the ingredients.
Step 5: Close the lid of the cooker and place the pipe in a tub containing cold water.
Step 6: Place the open end of the tube into a beaker.
Step 7: As the water heats up in the cooker, the steam containing oil passed through the tube.
Step 8: When this steam hits the cold water it turns into liquid and gets collected in the beaker.
Step 9: Once you are happy with the amount of oil collected, you can use a dropper to extract it and add to a sterilized glass jar.
Step 10: Place the jar in a cool, dark place for 2 days.

3. Infusion method

Infusion is the most cost effective and easiest method for the novice essential oil maker. There are a few simple steps for making your own infusion. Any herb or flower can be used. Choose something you love and will give you the most pleasure from making. The joy experienced from making and using your own essential oils can be healing in itself. It is easy to obtain herbs that are efficient in thyroid healing. Some examples include, rosemary, thyme or oregano, easily available in any grocery store or you can grow your own.

Step 1: Muddle your herb or herbs of choice.

Step 2: Put in a crock pot or double boiler.

Step 3: Fill with oil (grapeseed oil is recommended because it does not have a strong odor).

Step 4: Heat at a very low temperature (around 100 degrees) for around 5 hours.

Step 5: Strain your oil with cheesecloth (squeeze out all the excess) into an amber or cobalt blue jar and store in a cool, dark place like a cupboard.

Step 6: Enjoy for months to come!

Using essential oils

There are many ways in which essential oils can be used and some are as follows.

Inhalers:

Inhalers make for a good way to carry your essential oils around. An inhaler basically allows you to deeply inhale the essential oil such that it reaches the desired organs. An inhaler is a chapstick case that is inserted into the nostril and a big breath drawn in. It contains a piece of cotton, soaked with essential oil, contained inside a plastic tube. The tube has apertures on top that help the scent escape when drawn in. You can buy an inhaler or make one by yourself.

Diffusers:

Diffusers are devices that help release the essential oil into the atmosphere. A diffuser can be used to diffuse the aroma of the essential oil. The aroma of the essential oil helps release stress and anxiety and stimulates the pituitary gland.

Topical application:

The essential oil can also be applied topically in order to get relief from symptoms associated with the illness. Just a small drop of it applied over the area corresponding to thyroid gland can induce calm and control the symptoms to a large extent.

Daily regimen to use essential oils

Here is a simple everyday routine that you can follow.

Morning

As soon as you wake up in the morning, apply a little essential oil to your pulse points. This will help stimulate your senses and prepare you for the day ahead. You can also apply it over your thyroid region and wrap a warm cloth to help it penetrate better.

Afternoon

You can carry an inhaler to work so that it is easier to use as compared to applying topically. You can either buy an inhaler containing the right combination of oils or make one yourself. To do so, carefully open the inhaler and remove the piece of cotton contained within it. Prepare your combination of oils and dip a piece of cotton. You can also leave it to soak overnight. Gently squeeze and drop it inside the inhaler. Inhale every few hours to stimulate your thyroid gland. Replace the inhaler every 2 months or so.

Night

Make use of a diffuser at night to help you inhale the fragrance. There are many varieties of diffusers available in the market and you can use whatever you think will work well for you. Ensure that the diffuser is not too close to you as it can sometimes irritate your nasal passage. It is best to use a timed diffuser that goes off at preset times.

Reflexology refers to stimulating the pressure points on the body that are connected with the different organs. These pressure points lie under the feet and can be pressed to stimulate different organs and glands. For example, the top of the toe is connected to the brain and pressing it can help stimulate brain activity.

Similarly, the point just below it is pressed to stimulate the pituitary gland and can help regulate the TSH hormone. The area that lies just below the big toe corresponds with the thyroid gland. If you wish to stimulate your thyroid then you have to gently massage this area to relieve thyroid symptoms. Although reflexology can also be performed on the palm, it is much more effective below the feet.

It is best to use an essential oil like clove oil or a combination of oils to massage under the foot. Here is a recipe to try out.

20 drops basil

20 drops frankincense

20 drops myrrh

20 drops clove

20 drops lemongrass

20 drops marjoram

Add these to a small bottle filling the rest up with a carrier oil and give it a good shake. Use a little to place between your palms and rub together to heat it up. Massage it gently over the desired area. It will be important to do this on a daily basis in order to see substantial results.

Here are four ways in which you can incorporate reflexology into your daily routine.

Do it yourself

One of the best and simplest ways to get going is by learning the basics yourself and massaging your own feet. Thumb walking is a technique used in reflexology and can provide immense relief. Start by placing the tips of your thumbs over the chosen area and slowly walk them up and down. Apply a generous amount of oil on your palms and fingers so that they easily slide over the area.

Seek help

You can ask your partner, spouse, parent, sibling or friend to help you out. It can sometimes prove to be a better option, to let someone else do it as you will be able to sit back and relax. You can show them a video to teach them how it should be done or simply instruct them. Ensure that proper pressure is applied as too much or too little can cause discomfort.

Professional

You can visit a professional reflexologist. They will be aware of the various tips and tricks that can provide relief. They will also have a better understanding of the different points present under the foot and how best they can be stimulated.

Tools

There are many reflexology tools available that can be used to massage the foot. Some of them include rollers, acupressure tools etc. These will be easy to use and can serve to stimulate the thyroid.

Chapter 6
That Stuff Burns my Skin!
(or Essential Oils Safety)

Buying Essential Oils

When it comes to buying essential oils, you have to bear in mind a few criteria that will help you pick out the best. Here they are in detail.

Quality
The first priority should be given to quality. It is vital to look for good quality essential oils that have been prepared using quality ingredients. You have to look for labels that say "100% organic, 100% pure, therapeutic grade". These indicate the quality of the product and make it ideal for people to use for therapeutic purposes. The ones you buy should be free from chemicals and contain 100% pure essential oils. In order to ensure a higher purity of an oil it is important to obtain the gas chromatography-mass spectrometry (GC-MS) report from the vendor. There should be a new GC-MS report with each batch or lot and it should be dated, with the lot number on the report and the bottle of essential oil that came from that batch matching. This should be considered along with making sure it is organic or wild-crafted, if possible, and sourced from the countries that it grows indigenously.

Price
If you are buying them in bulk then look for combination packs. These will be priced lesser than single packs and can

be used in combination with each other. Good quality oils will be priced higher than low-quality ones.

Specialty stores
Specialty online stores will sell high-quality oils as compared to drugstores or even health food stores. It is difficult to find truly high quality oils and some labels can be misleading and claim they are the best when this is not the case. The following are some suggestions, from Kurt Schnaubelt, for websites/places to find high quality, authentic, unadulterated essential oils.
Websites:
www.labofflowers.com
www.naturesgift.com
www.originalswissaromatics.com
www.whitelotusaromatics.com
Physical address:
Ron Guba
39 Melverton Drive
Hallam, VICTORIA 3803
Australia
Ph: 03 8795 720

Safe Use
When considering using an essential oil on your body it is important to know the safety guidelines with that specific oil and also know how it reacts with you personally. When you purchase a new oil, ensure you conduct a patch test. This means you apply a small quantity on the inside of your elbow to test if it suits your skin. If you develop rashes, you could be allergic to that specific oil and it is best not to use it. The safety precautions are different for each oil, some are more irritant than others. A good rule of thumb is not to ingest them unless you have thoroughly researched the safe use and consulted with someone with extensive experience and education in essential oils. With topical usage of oils, it

is best to dilute the oil with a carrier oil like fractionated coconut oil, almond oil, grapeseed oil, etc.

Chapter 7
Do I Have To??
(or Diet, Exercise and Homeopathy)

Diet Tips

Ensure that you consume timely meals. Set schedules so that you eat your meals on time. It is important to get rid of gluten from your diet. It will worsen hypothyroidism and can lead to Hashimoto's.

You might have to consume supplements to help your body cope with thyroid issues. Selenium is one such supplement that is highly recommended to those with autoimmune diseases. Yellow fin tuna, sardines, grass-fed beef, turkey, beef liver, chicken and spinach are all some of the foods that are rich in selenium and can be used to relieve Hashimoto symptoms. Brazil nuts and eggs are also rich in selenium, but can cause problems in people with Hashimoto's or other autoimmune diseases.

Omega 3 fatty acids should be a big part of your diet. It helps in controlling thyroid function. Freshwater fish such as salmon and trout make good choices. Be sure that it reads "wild caught" on the label as this will ensure that there are fewer toxins, especially heavy metals. You can also consume omega 3 supplements.

Vitamin D is a nutrient that helps in enhancing thyroid function. According to studies, a majority of people suffer from vitamin D deficiency. One good way of fixing this is by spending time under the sun. Play a sport and try to get under the sun as much as possible. You can also consume a vitamin D3 after consulting a physician.

Apart from essential oils, there are also a few herbs that are full of goodness. Some of these include Bacopa, ginseng, ashwagandha and dandelion. You can consume supplements containing these herbs or their extracts.

Increase your intake of green, leafy vegetables. Anything from spinach to kale to broccoli, try to consume at least one green vegetable per day as this will increase your magnesium intake and many are deficient in this very important nutrient. A note of caution on the green and leafy vegetables mentioned; they cruciferous vegetables which are known to contain goitrogens which have been thought to cause problems with your thyroid, but it is not conclusive. Cooking these vegetables will decrease their goitrogen content. You must also increase vitamin A content and consume those vegetables and fruits that are rich in this particular nutrient. Try not to overcook the vegetables and focus on making smoothies and salads out of them. It is a good practice to use organic, raw and unrefined extra virgin coconut oil for cooking. It is light on the body and heats up at a higher temperature.

It is quite important to check your water content. Some water can be high in salts that can affect your thyroid function. You must drink filtered water to prevent any chemicals and chlorine from entering your body.

Gently detox on a regular basis in order to get rid of any built-up chemicals and salts in your body. There are many ways in which you can detox including taking sauna baths, drinking smoothies, exercising etc. You can also do Pilates as this helps control thyroid function.

These form the dietary and lifestyle tips to follow in order to enhance thyroid function.

Exercise

Exercise is one of the most important aspects of life. It is vital for people to work out every day, especially those with a thyroid issue.

Here are some pointers for the same.

#1: Try to exercise every day. Follow a set schedule so that you don't miss a single day of exercise.

#2: If you are not motivated enough to take up exercising then consider joining a gym. You will find it easier to take up physical activity, especially if you employ a physical trainer.

#3: Start slow if you are not accustomed to exercising. Taking on too much at once can sometimes make it difficult for your body to process the changes.

#4: Ask a partner to join in so that you feel motivated to take it up seriously.

#5: Set yourself weight loss goals and work towards it. Measure your progress every few weeks to remain inspired.

#6: Reward yourself from time to time. It will keep you inspired to keep going.

#7: When it comes to improving thyroid function, you require rigorous exercises that can stimulate the gland. Simple ones such as Pilates will not do the trick and can only be taken up as supplementary exercises.

#8: Following are some basic thyroid stimulating exercises.

Cardio Exercises

Cardio exercises happen to be one of the best thyroid enhancing exercises to follow. Cardio exercises get your heart rate up and force your body to up the pace. Your glands and organs feel energized and start functioning optimally. There are many types of cardio exercises to choose from including swimming, running, jogging etc.

Mix it up so that you do not get bored of the routine. Swimming is particularly a great exercise to consider as you will not feel as stressed and still manage to stimulate your organs.

Aerobics

Aerobics is another great option, especially for women looking to enhance thyroid function. Aerobics is a form of dance exercise that is fun to take up. You can either join an aerobics class or watch videos while exercising. Take up those exercises that are known to affect the thyroid positively. Try to mix it up with regular dancing so that it doesn't get monotonous.

Cross-fit Training

Cross fit training is a type of interval training that involves taking up rigorous exercises followed by a small break. Alternate between the two until your body feels the burn. There are many predetermined sets to choose from and can pick whatever suits your body best.

HIIT

High intensity interval training (HIIT) is recommended as the best exercise for thyroid patients and also works most efficiently in weight loss. This form of exercise causes the least stress on the body and it takes less time to get results, therefore it is very efficient and works well for those with busy schedules. It gets your heart rate up and blood flowing very quickly and can be implemented in aerobics training and weight training. 20 to 40 minutes a day is all that is needed. The basic idea for HIIT is that you will train in intervals of activity and rest. The active intervals are highly intense, meaning they will have you breathing very heavily. For instance, if you sprinted for 30 to 60 seconds. The resting intervals are your recovery and it is recommended that you listen to your body. The rest time will usually be the same as the active time or more, depending on what you need.

Don't forget to warm up before exercising so that your body is able to absorb the exercise.

Homeopathy

Homeopathy can be another powerful natural strategy for treating thyroid symptoms and it can be used along with aromatherapy. Although it is important to use caution especially when employing aromatherapy because there can be essential oils that are not efficient to use with certain homeopathic remedies because they can block their action. Mainly peppermint, chamomile and essential oils with a high camphor content can antidote certain homeopathic treatments. Peppermint blocks the action of those from the Natrum family (Nat. Mur., Nat. Phos., etc.)[xv]

The concept of homeopathic treatment is very similar to the idea of vaccinations or immunizations because it uses a substance that causes the symptoms of a disease to cure the disease, but in very small amounts, although the difference is that homeopathy is natural and so diluted that it may not contain any molecule of the actual substance. Also, a goal of homeopathy is not to try to suppress symptoms, but to treat the individual person and the entire body to create balance and to minimize susceptibility to disease. There are many homeopathic treatments that can be used for thyroid conditions and the different effects of a thyroid condition. An obvious possible option is the homeopathic treatment called Thyroidinum.

Chapter 8
What Do I Do Now?
(or Putting it all together)

Step 1: Find a functional medicine practitioner who is open to natural methods. You can find this type of doctor in your area by going to www.functionalmedicine.org.

Step 2: Get your thyroid tested through a blood test. Pamela Wartian Smith advocates adding a free T3 & T4 and rT3 test to the conventional set of factors tested to determine thyroid function. She lists an example test interpretation in her book about thyroid disorders. The normal range may vary from lab to lab.

Test: TSH
Normal Range: 0.3 to 2.0
Possible Diagnosis:
High TSH indicates an underactive thyroid (hypothyroidism)
Low TSH indicates an overactive thyroid (hyperthyroidism)
Test: Free T4
Normal Range: 0.7 to 2.0
Possible Diagnosis:
Levels are low (hypothyroidism)
Levels are elevated (hyperthyroidism)
Test: Free T3
Normal Range: 2.3 to 4.2
Possible Diagnosis:

Levels are low (hypothyroidism)

Levels are elevated (hyperthyroidism)

Test: rT3

Possible Diagnosis:

Levels elevated (triggered by chronic stress, pneumonia, injury, surgery, low-iron, or low-cortisol) (hypothyroidism or hyperthyroidism)

Thyroid antibodies:

Test: Antithyroglobulin

Normal Range: Negative

Possible Diagnosis:

Positive indicates Hashimoto's thyroiditis

Test: Antimicrosomal

Normal Range: Negative

Possible Diagnosis:

Positive indicates Hashimoto's thyroiditis, autoimmune hemolytic anemia, Graves' disease, Sjogren syndrome, systemic lupus erythematosus, rheumatoid arthritis, and/or thyroid cancer

Test: Antithyroperoxidase

Normal Range: Negative

Possible Diagnosis:

Positive indicates Hashimoto's thyroiditis, Graves' disease, Sjogren's syndrome, lupus, rheumatoid arthritis, and/or pernicious anemia[xvi]

Step 3: Find an aromatherapist with extensive training in essential oils and aromatherapy healing. You can do this by going to https://naha.org/find-an-aromatherapist.

Step 4: Decide which essential oils and methods will benefit you the most from the description. If you are strapped for cash, there's nothing wrong with starting with only 1 or 2 and gradually building your stash. Roller bottles are your best friend! And labels. Become a mixologist and get mixin'. A great general blend to start with for stress and deep breathing includes equal parts cajeput, clove bud oil, clary sage and ylang ylang used with fractionated coconut oil as a carrier oil.

Step 5: Come up with an easy exercise routine that is quick and you won't have a problem sticking to. Circuit training is something you don't need any equipment for and can provide beneficial results in as little as 10 to 20 minutes a few days a week

Step 6: Come up with a meal plan that fits your lifestyle and what your body needs.

Step 7: Make it a point to pray and meditate on a daily basis. Prayer helps you connect with your Maker, who is your Ultimate Source of love. You will get to know your true purpose through prayer and this will lead to true fulfillment. There are also studies that have determined that prayer lowers your stress levels. Try to pray and meditate for as long as you can everyday. Listen in the "classroom of silence," as Matthew Kelly refers to it.

Step 8: Just do it!

Conclusion

Thank you again for purchasing this book! I hope the information contained here was able to help you in finding relief and open the door to healing for your thyroid symptoms. The next step is to implement your aromatherapy plan for health and happiness.

It will require a certain amount of dedication but give way to positive results. I hope you are able to put into practice all that you read in this book.

Lastly, if you were pleased with this book and it helped you in some way, then allow me to request your support. Would you be gracious enough to submit a review for this book on Amazon? I would truly appreciate it! I also welcome any suggestions on how this book can be improved or suggestions for other types of information to include.

Please submit a review for this book on Amazon!

Thank you and God bless you on your journey!

Other books in the Thyroid Health Series

Fermentation and Thyroid Health: Anxious? Bloated? Sluggish? Get Relief with Over 20 Fermented Food Recipes to Help Heal Your Thyroid

References

[i]http://hypothyroidmom.com/the-two-big-problems-with-typical-thyroid-hormone-treatment-part-1-of-2/

[ii]http://hypothyroidmom.com/the-two-big-problems-with-typical-thyroid-hormone-treatment-part-2-of-2/

[iii]https://www.hashimotoshealing.com/5-keys-improving-thyroid-hormone-conversion/

[iv]Schnaubelt, Kurt. *The Healing Intelligence of Essential Oils: The Science of Advanced Aromatherapy.* Rochester, Toronto: Healing Arts Press, 2011. Print.

[v]Davis, Patricia. *Aromatherapy: An A-Z: The most comprehensive guide to aromatherapy ever published.* London: Vermillion, 2005. Print.

[vi]http://drjockers.com/10-tips-boost-dhea-levels/

[vii]http://roberttisserand.com/2010/11/the-oxygenation-myth/

[viii]https://www.restartmed.com/increase-free-t3-naturally/

[ix]https://draxe.com/diabetic-diet-plan/

[x]https://www.ncbi.nlm.nih.gov/pmc/articles/PMC2901047/

[xi]https://www.ncbi.nlm.nih.gov/pubmed/24802524

[xii]https://www.ncbi.nlm.nih.gov/pubmed/10082788

[xiii]http://www.jfda-online.com/article/S1021-9498(14)00059-3/pdf

[xiv]https://www.ncbi.nlm.nih.gov/pubmed/2985357

[xv]Schnaubelt, Kurt. *The Healing Intelligence of Essential Oils: The Science of Advanced Aromatherapy.* Rochester, Toronto: Healing Arts Press, 2011. Print.

[xvi]Wartian Smith, MD, MPH, Pamela. *What You Must Know About Thyroid Disorders and What to do About Them.* Garden City Park: Square One Publishers, 2016. Print.